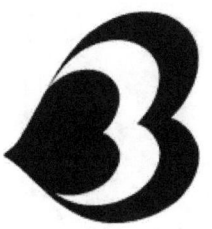

52

INSPIRATIONS

FOR HEALTHY

Loving Couples

52 QUESTIONS FOR A HEALTHY LOVING COUPLES

DEDICATION

I dedicate this book to my loving husband Vincent. I would have never known the true meaning of love without you. You are my inspiration every day to love myself first and then share this beautiful love with the world! Thank you for all your love!

INTRODUCTION

This simple book is designed to help you build a stronger and healthier relationship with yourself and your partner.

As a personal trainer and group fitness instructor I work with wonderful couples every day. I wrote this book to give you and those couples simple ways to deepen their health and their relationships.

You can choose an inspiration anywhere in the book and share it with your partner whenever you please. Each activity is designed to be simple and fun and I really hope you enjoy them.

I have also left blank space to the left of each inspiration for you to add notes and thoughts from your conversations.

Have fun and enjoy your relationship!

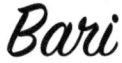

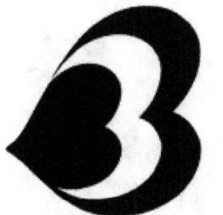

Take a walk holding hands

Give a genuine smile to your partner

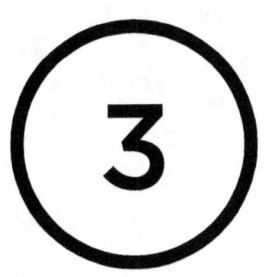

Cook something simple together

Sit outside together

Extra Credit:
Sit in a Hammock!

Go to bed at the same time

Ask your partner what a perfect day would look like

Say one thing
your partner
is doing
really well

Breathe deeply and consciously listen to your partner

Do a morning stretch together

Share one thing you loved about your partner the first time you saw them

Practice great posture today

Extra Credit:
Try balancing a book on your head for 5 minutes

Go smell the roses somewhere together

When you're hungry today drink water first

Say one thing you are grateful about to your partner

Play ball with your partner inside or outside

Hug your partner as soon as you see them at the end of the day

10 Surprising Benefits of Hugs:
Flip to the resources at the back for more

Say one encouraging thing to your partner

Go on
a hike
together

Notice one beautiful thing about your partner

Grill something outside together

Surprise your partner with a glass of water

Pay attention to your deep love for your partner when you next look at them

Turn off the TV and celebrate eating together

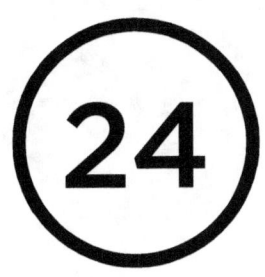

Create a nighttime routine you love

Do 25 jumping jacks with your partner

Bonus Points:
Research shows 50 hops prevents osteoporosis

Try a five minute meditation together

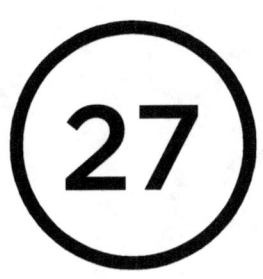

Have a picnic with your sweetheart

Talk about a treasured memory you both have

Drink a glass of water first thing when you wake up

Set personal time aside each for other often

Surprise your partner with a short local trip

Research each other's heritage and traditions

Set aside quality time during the week to be together

Write a love note to your partner

Share two of
your partner's
positive
characteristics
that you love

Talk about your optimistic future together

Give each other the gift of patience

Make a colorful meal together

Do what you
do best and let
your partner
do what they
do best

Hide a love note in your partner's gym bag

Make a hot cup of tea for your loved one

Sign up for a class together

Remember to love yourself first

Share one thing you've learned during the day with your lover

Make a list of three of your favorite exercises

Plan an escape together

Go swimming in nature

Do five minutes of simple stretches with your partner

Play and be playful - do something silly together

Watch a documentary on love together

Hike a mountain and find out where a trail leads to together

Encourage each other while exercising

RESOURCES

10

SURPRISING BENEFITS OF HUGS

1. **Trust** : A nurturing hug builds trust and a sense of safety. This helps with open and honest communication.

2. **Healing** : Hugs can instantly boost oxytocin levels, which heal feelings of loneliness, isolation, and anger.

3. **Serotonin** : Holding a hug for an extended time lifts one's serotonin levels, elevating mood and creating happiness.

4. **Immunity** : Hugs strengthen the immune system. The gentle pressure on the sternum and the emotional charge this creates activates the thymus gland, which regulates and balances the body's production of white blood cells, which keep you healthy.

5. **Self-Esteem** : Since we were little touch showed us that we're loved and special. These tactile sensations from our early years are still embedded in our nervous system as adults. The cuddles we received growing up remain imprinted at a cellular level and hugs remind us of that at a somatic level. Hugs, therefore, connect us to our ability to self love.

6. **Relaxation** : Hugging relaxes muscles. Hugs release tension in the body. Hugs can take away pain; they soothe aches by increasing circulation into the soft tissues.

7. **Balance** : Hugs balance out the nervous system. The galvanic skin response of someone receiving and giving a hug shows a change in skin conductance. The effect in moisture and electricity in the skin suggests a more balanced state in the para-sympathetic nervous system.

8. **Giving** : Hugs teach us how to give and receive. There is equal value in receiving and being receptive to warmth, as to giving and sharing. Hugs educate us how love flows both ways.

9. **Be Present** : Hugs are much like meditation and laughter. They teach us to let go and be present in the moment. They encourage us to flow with the energy of life. Hugs get you out of your circular thinking patterns and connect you with your heart and your feelings and your breath.

10. **Relationships** : The exchange between people hugging is an investment in the relationship. It encourages empathy and understanding. And, it's synergistic, which means the whole is more than the sum of its parts. This synergy is more likely to result in win-win outcomes.

ABOUT THE AUTHOR

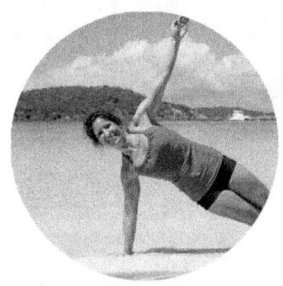

Bari Ramirez is a certified personal trainer and group fitness instructor and is the owner of Body by Bari.

She leads trainings and classes in and around Woodstock, Vermont where she lives with her loving husband. Her mission is to be happy as a positive role model through wellness as she supports and educates her clients.

52 Inspirations for Healthy Loving Couples is her first book.

To work with Bari and explore her online classes please visit her expanding library at BodybyBari.com.

ABOUT THE EDITOR

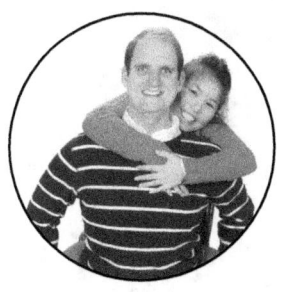

Travis Hellstrom is a leadership coach, professor and author who loves helping people lead happy and simple lives.

He also loves writing books and sharing them with the world with incredible friends like Bari. He counts himself lucky to be one of the many people inspired by her passion and dedication.

Travis is the author of the *Peace Corps Volunteer's Handbook*, *Questions for the Dalai Lama*, *52 Questions for a Better Relationship* and several other books.

To find them and read more from Travis visit: TravisHellstrom.com.